ELLA HUBBLE

Skin Care for Dry Skin

A holistic guide for dry, ichthyosis, and eczema prone skin

I want to dedicate this book to my beloved mother, Rasathi, the kindest person I have ever known. She has supported my skin journey since childhood, always showered me kindly with love, and taught me to love my skin.

I would like also to dedicate this book to everyone with a skin condition.

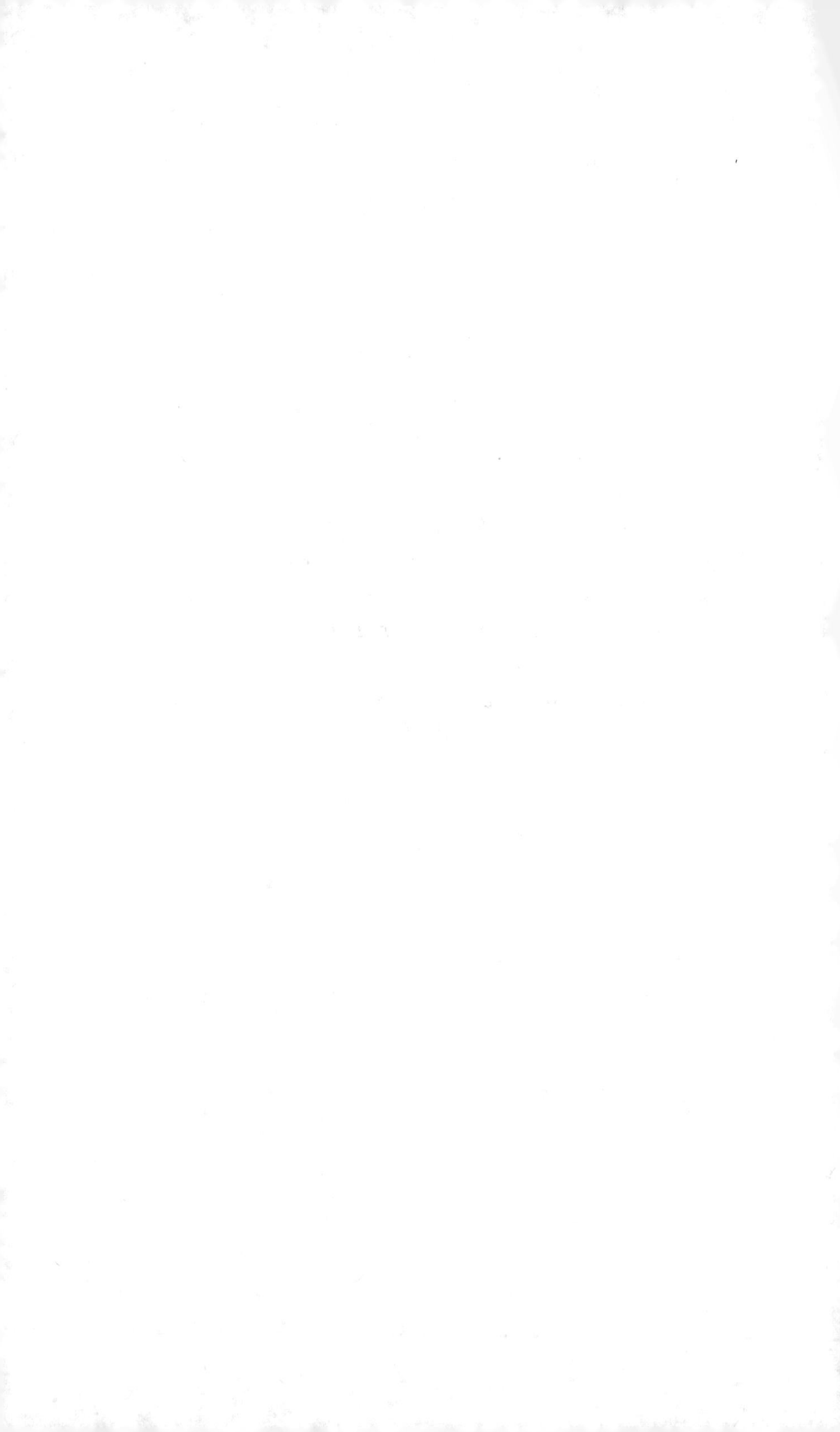

Our skin, the body's largest organ,
deserves nothing less than the largest
measure of our love

-Ella Hubble

Contents

1

Introduction

In my early twenties, I was diagnosed with a rare skin condition, ichthyosis vulgaris. This pivotal moment set me on a path of self-discovery and empowerment. I have dehydrated skin, which is also eczema-prone. This diagnosis was a turning point, allowing me to educate, understand, and manage my skin. Understanding your skin condition is the first step towards taking control of your skin health. This journey of self-discovery and empowerment is not just mine, but it's a path that you can also embark on, leading to a better understanding and management of your skin health.

At around eight years old, I remember going to my GP doctor with my mother and asking the doctor why I had wrinkled hands at this age. I requested an antidote to straighten out my wrinkles. His response disappointed me when there was no 'magic' cream, and he prescribed me aqueous cream instead. This cream mildly helped to hydrate my skin briefly before it was back to being scaly. People would often comment on my 'wooden' hand. No number of creams or moisturisers worked on my hands. Besides my face and neck, my entire body was dehydrated. My skin was scaly and flaky, and people would sometimes comment on my skin, referring to it as 'snake-like' and 'cracked.' Over-the-counter dry skin creams did not particularly help with my skin. I was on a mission to find a cure.

My dry skin conditions, particularly during my teenage years, presented numerous challenges. I dreaded physical education and swimming lessons, often needing to be collected by my mother for lunch at home so I could apply the cream before swimming. In secondary school, I even avoided these lessons altogether. The insensitivity of some students towards my skin was hurtful. I overheard them referring to me as having 'granny' skin or being 'dry.' These experiences often left me feeling deeply insecure about my skin, leading to hours, days, and nights of overthinking and tears.

One sunny weekend, my grandad lost conscientiousness, and I was in the ambulance taking him to the hospital. Besides the dramatic scenery, my grandad was thankfully well and fine. The doctors discharged my grandad after a day, and they did not seem too concerned about his medical needs, but they were more startled by his skin, and we came home with bottles of prescribed creams. It was on this day that I came to a realisation that my grandad has ichthyosis vulgaris, and it is hereditary. He also had asthma, which is another sign as people often with dry skin have other co-occurring symptoms. It has skipped a whole generation; my mother's skin is soft and smooth, and I have inherited ichthyosis vulgaris, eczema, asthma, and allergies.

My quest for healthier, more hydrated skin led to extensive

research and various solutions to manage my ichthyosis vulgaris and eczema. Sharing my findings can benefit a larger community of individuals struggling with dry skin. I discovered that considering both internal and external factors, a holistic approach was the most effective way to manage my condition. While there may not be a cure for inherited dry skin, there are numerous ways to manage it effectively. This management must be approached holistically, considering both internal and external factors. It requires a lifestyle change to find clarity and understand your skin's unique story.

Skin journal

How would I describe my skin type and condition?

....
....
....
....
....

Do I recall an early memory of noticing or thinking about my skin?

....
....
....
....
....

....
......

How did this make me feel? Has this impacted me growing up? ....
....
....
....
....
....
....
....

Are there any skin-related conditions in my family history?

....
....
....
....
....

How are my feelings and relationship with my skin today?

....
....
....
....
....
....
......

What would I say to my younger self?

....

....

....

....

....

....

......

What are my skin goals?

....

....

....

....

....

2

The importance of skincare for dry skin

The skin is the largest organ of the human body. The skin is a good indicator of your general health and a direct reflection of your inner health. The medical term for dry skin is xeroderma, and for dehydrated skin is Xerosis. Dry skin occurs when your body is unable to retain moisture. Normal skin owes its soft and pliable texture to its water content; it can keep the water. To help protect against water loss, the outer layer of the skin produces an oily substance, sebum. If the oil is depleted, the skin becomes dry. Dry skin is a common condition affecting individuals of all ages and skin types. Due to the lack of moisture, it presents with symptoms such as scaliness, tightness, itching, and sometimes cracks. A sound skincare routine is essential to maintain skin health and alleviate discomfort.

Maintaining Skin Barrier Function: A skincare routine is vital for dry skin to maintain the skin's barrier function. The outermost layer of the skin, the stratum corneum, acts as a barrier that protects it from external factors such as UV radiation, pollutants, and germs. With dry skin, the outer layer doesn't produce enough oil and sebum, which makes the skin more prone to damage. A skincare routine focusing on moisturising and hydrating helps strengthen the skin barrier, keeping it resilient.

Prevent Premature Ageing: Dry skin is more prone to premature ageing through wrinkles, fine lines, and sagging. When your skin lacks moisture and hydration, it can appear rough, dull, and aged. Hydrating your skin can help prevent premature ageing and maintain a youthful glow. Moisturisers and treatments that focus on hydration and anti-aging properties can improve the overall texture and appearance of the skin.

Boosting Confidence and Self-Esteem: You may continuously or at some point feel insecure about your dry skin. It may affect your choice of clothing and your socialising with others. With a proper skincare routine, your skin's texture and complexion will improve, and you will feel more confident in your skin, contributing to a positive self-image.

Enhancing Skin Health: A skincare routine is essential for healthy skin overall. Dry skin is more prone to conditions such as eczema and ichthyosis, which I will expand on in the upcoming chapters. Having a targeted skincare routine is, therefore, essential. It will help promote healthy skin and alleviate discomfort and irritation. Ingredients like aloe vera, hyaluronic acid, and ceramides have calming and hydrating properties that relieve dry, irritated skin.

Therefore, it is crucial to have a skincare routine for dry skin. This is not only for cosmetic reasons but also for maintaining overall skin health and confidence in your skin. It is about owning your skin and feeling empowered. Investing your time and effort in a consistent, tailored skincare routine will give you long-term benefits and improved skin quality. A good skincare routine is a powerful tool in your journey towards healthier, more comfortable skin.

3

Identifying the dry skin condition

Understanding your type of dry skin condition is of high importance. It will help you to tailor your skincare for more focused and targeted help. It will help you understand your skin's needs and help develop an effective treatment plan. Genetics, environmental conditions, and certain medical conditions can cause dry skin. See if any family members have a similar skin texture or any allergies commonly associated with dry skin. Stay intuitive and listen to your body if external factors, such as harsh soaps, are drying your skin. There are many dry skin conditions, such as psoriasis, but I will focus on eczema and ichthyosis vulgaris.

What is eczema?

Eczema, or dermatitis, is a non-contagious, inflammatory, dry skin condition characterised by inflamed, red, and dry, itchy skin. It is often seen in individuals with a family history of allergies or asthma and can occur at any age.

There are many types of eczema, each with different triggers: atopic dermatitis, contact dermatitis, dyshidrotic, neurodermatitis, nummular eczema, and seborrheic dermatitis.

Establishing a good skincare routine is important, but it is also essential to identify and avoid triggers that cause your eczema to flare. There is no cure for genetically inherited eczema; however, you have control and influence over your environment and stress level. The goal is to reduce discomfort and prevent infection and flare-ups.

Symptoms

Intense Itching: It is a hallmark symptom and can be severe, leading to scratching, bleeding of the skin, and potential skin damage.

Dryness and Flaking: Tends to be parched, rough, and flaky, especially during flare-ups.

Red, inflamed skin: The appearance can be reddish and inflamed patches.

Blisters and Oozing: In severe cases, it can lead to the formation of blisters that may ooze fluid.

Characteristics

Atopic dermatitis: A form of atopic dermatitis which is associated with allergies and hypersensitive immune response.

Triggers: Flare-ups can be triggered by a range of factors, including allergens such as dust mites and pollen, stress, irritants, and environmental conditions such as the weather (cold climate, which can dry the skin).

Chronic: It is chronic and recurrent, with periods of flare-ups.

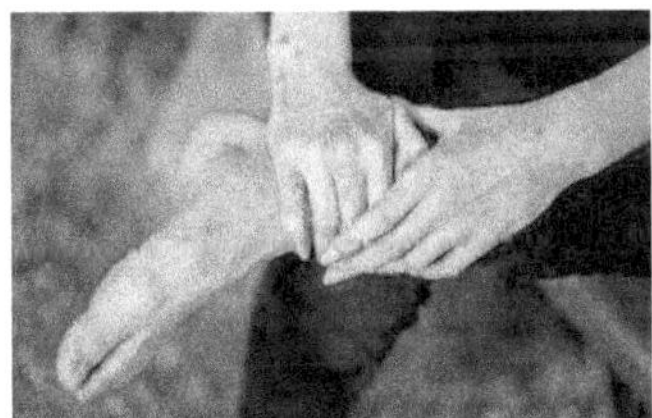 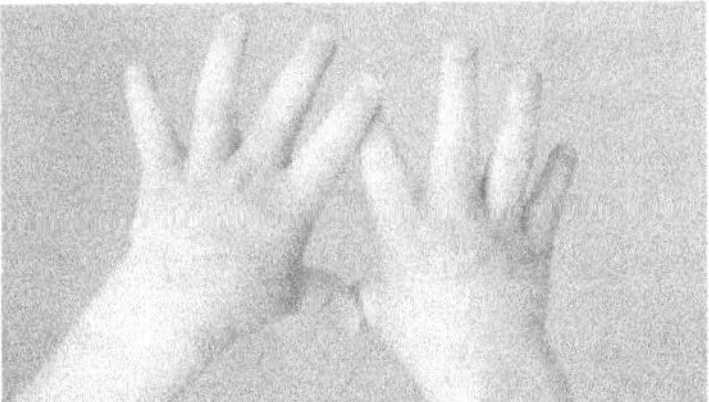

What is ichthyosis vulgaris?

'Ichthyosis' is a group of skin conditions characterised by dry, scaly skin. Ichthyosis vulgaris is the most common form of inherited ichthyosis, and this is what I will be discussing. This skin appears to be dry and flaky with the build-up of scales in certain areas, usually the outer part of the lower legs, arms, and abdomen. The palms and soles have noticeably more wrinkles on the skin, regardless of your age.

There are many different types of ichthyosis, such as lamellar,

X-linked, and harlequin ichthyosis, and it is essential that you find out what type you may have to get targeted help.

There is no cure for ichthyosis, but establishing a good skincare routine is vital to managing the symptoms. The goal is to improve the skin's condition by reducing the scales and hydrating it to relieve discomfort.

Symptoms

Dry, scaly skin: 'Fish-like' scales and texture are due to the thickened, dry, and flaky skin.

Increased Skin Line: Increased and profound, especially on the palms of the hand and soles of the feet. Wrinkled skin.

Affected Areas: It can affect specific areas of the body, usually the outer area of the legs and arms, or be more generalised, covering large areas of the skin.

Characteristics

Genetic Condition: It is often inherited and passed down through families.

Autosomal Dominant Inheritance: In most cases, a child only needs to inherit one copy of the defective gene to develop the condition.

Chronic: It is a chronic condition but can be managed with skincare and lifestyle modifications.

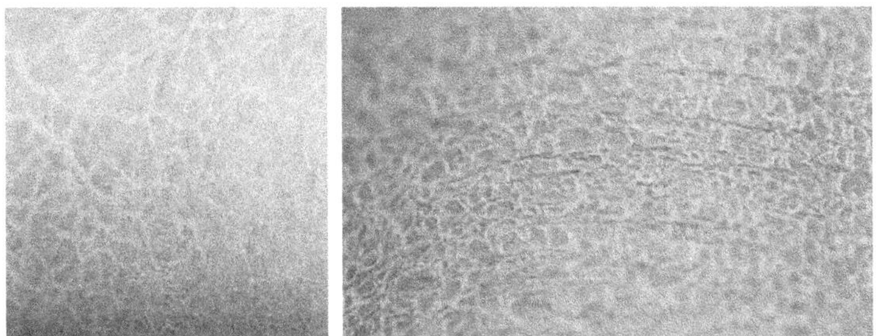

4

Moisturising skin from within

A holistic approach beyond a skincare routine is crucial to maintaining healthy skin. This involves nourishing your skin from within with nutrition and hydration. It is a lifestyle change. I have gathered some changes to benefit those with dry skin conditions.

Dry Skin Friendly Food: Food rich in Omega-3 fatty acids, such as salmon, mackerel, flaxseeds, and chia seeds, can help reduce inflammation. Antioxidant-rich foods such as dark leafy greens like spinach and kale, berries such as blueberries, and nuts protect the skin from oxidative stress and promote skin repair. Food rich in vitamins and minerals such as vitamins A, C, E, and zinc. It plays a crucial role in skin health and wound healing. This includes carrots, pumpkin seeds, and citrus fruits. Maintain a balanced diet rich in whole foods like fruits, vegetables, lean proteins, and healthy fats like avocado. Probiotics such as yogurt are good for gut health and maintaining healthy skin.

Hydration: Drink plenty of water to keep your skin hydrated. It will maintain skin moisture and health. Aim to drink a minimum of 8 glasses of water per day. Adding a piece of fruit to the water can add a hint of flavour. Hydrating beverages such as coconut water are rich in electrolytes that help maintain skin hydration.

Avoid Food Sensitivities: People with certain dry skin conditions, such as eczema, often have triggers to certain foods. It is essential that you find your triggers and any intolerances or allergies. Keeping a food diary can help with this, and allergy and intolerance tests can also be used. Once identified, these foods should be avoided as they can cause flare-ups and skin inflammation. Typical food triggers include gluten, dairy, and processed food. Avoid processed and excessive sugar, which can contribute to skin inflammation.

Limit dehydrating foods and drinks: Try to reduce the consumption of alcohol, which will dehydrate and further exacerbate the skin. Avoid caffeinated beverages, which have a diuretic effect and can lead to dehydration. Avoid buying drinks high in sugar.

Herbal teas and supplements: Herbal teas such as green tea and chamomile have anti-inflammatory and antioxidant properties that benefit skin health. Some supplements can help maintain good skin health. Contact your healthcare provider or dermatologist about incorporating skin-supporting supplements such as Vitamin D, cod liver oil, and probiotics into your daily routine.

Self-Journal

Hydration

How much water did I drink today? *Reflect on whether you met your hydration goals and if you notice any changes in your skin's texture*

....

....

Did I notice a difference in my skin's hydration on days I drank more water? *Look for signs such as plumpness, less tightness, or reduced flakiness?*

....

....

How does my skin feel immediately after drinking water throughout the day? *Do you notice any immediate or gradual changes in how hydrated it feels?*

....

....

Diet

What did I eat today, and did I notice any impact on my skin? *List any salty, processed, or sugary foods and observe if these correlate with increased dryness.*

....

....

Did I include any foods known to support skin health? *List any vegetables, fruits, and nuts.*

....

....

Did I consume any caffeinated drinks today? *Note if caffeine seems to affect your skin's moisture levels, especially if you feel more dehydrated afterward.*

....

....

Have I noticed any positive effects from certain foods, like avocados, fish, nuts, or seeds, on my skin? *Track if these omega-rich foods seem to improve hydration over time.*

....

....

Have I made any changes to my diet recently and have these affected my skin? *Note any new foods or eliminated items and observe if there's a noticeable change.*

....

....

5

Skincare routine for dry skin

Incorporating a daily skincare regime and selecting products tailored to your dry skin type can improve, protect, and maintain skin health. Here are some external considerations for the skin.

Exfoliation: Exfoliate your skin with a gentle exfoliant to remove dead skin cells and promote skin renewal. Avoid hard scrubs, which can irritate or damage dry skin. Removal of scales can be aided by keratolytic, such as moisturisers with salicylic acid, which helps dissolve the scales. This improves the appearance of the skin and allows creams to penetrate the skin. Pairing this routine with an exfoliant mitt will help scrub off the sales build-up. It is particularly beneficial for those with ichthyosis vulgaris, as there is a build of scales.

Hydrating Moisturisers: Choose thick, emollient-rich creams that provide long-lasting hydration and lock in moisturise. Always moisturize your skin immediately after bathing or showering to seal in moisture. Oat-based moisturisers are beneficial for eczema-prone skin and have anti-inflammatory properties.

With Ichthyosis vulgaris, creams with alpha-hydroxy acids, such as lactic acids, effectively hydrate the skin. Look for products containing hyaluronic acid or glycerine, which attract and retain moisture in the skin. Ingredients like petrolatum or shea butter help to create a protective barrier on the skin and prevent moisture loss.

Hypoallergenic Products and Avoid Irritants: Choose gentle, fragrance-free cleansers or mild soap-free cleansers that will not strip skin of natural oils. Choose alcohol-free Products, as alcohol can be drying and exacerbate dry skin issues. Hypoallergenic products are those catered for sensitive skin and formulated to be less likely to cause allergic reactions. Opt for products that are hypoallergenic.

Shower, Bathing, and Pat Dry: Avoid hot water, which can further dry the skin. When washing your face and body, opt for lukewarm water. Soft water has been treated to remove "hard" minerals like calcium and magnesium. It's much better for your skin since it does not contain minerals that strip away moisture or block your pores. Unfortunately, the water from the tap is not treated, and it can be costly to install soft water. Depending on the severity of your dry skin condition and individual circumstances, installing water can be an investment in your skin. Pat dry with a soft towel after your shower so you are gentle on the skin and prevent from further irritation.

Overnight Treatments: Moisturise hands and feet. Apply a thick moisturiser to your hands and feet before bed, and wear cotton gloves or socks to lock in moisture overnight. Urea based products will be effective for cracked heels. Cracked heels and fissures are familiar with ichthyosis vulgaris. This is a great nightly routine for moisturising feet.

Sun Protection and Clothing: Apply a minimum of SPF 30 sunscreen to protect skin from sun damage and prevent further dryness. Wear protective clothing such as sunglasses and a sunhat to avoid further sun damage. Wool and synthetic materials such as nylon and polyester cause overheating, sweating, and irritation, exacerbating itchy skin. 100% cotton is a desirable choice for eczema sufferers. The loose material doesn't aggravate the skin and lets it breathe easily.

Seeking Professional Health: Contact a dermatologist if you have persistent or severe symptoms that may benefit from a diagnosis for a targeted intervention. They will be able to personalise a treatment plan and provide recommendations. They may also offer prescription-based medications and creams unavailable in stores to effectively manage your dry skin condition.

My personal recommendation for ichthyosis vulgaris skin is to use **G16 Skin Repair**

Lotion. It is formulated to eliminate dead skin cells and encourages the production of new, healthy cells, resulting in a glowing and nourished complexion. It penetrates deeply into the skin to repair the underlying layers before they reach the surface. Once the G16 lotion course is completed, a chosen daily moisturiser will work best. I personally find Aveeno moisturising lotion works well for dehydrated and sensitive skin.

When eczema flares up, it is good to contact the doctor. Prescribed steroids reduce the inflammation of the eczema. Your doctor needs to prescribe and consult this first.

Self-Journal

Sensitivities

Did my skin feel irritated or extra dry after using specific products or ingredients today? *Note any cleansers, creams, or serums and their effects.*

....

....

Did I encounter any potential irritants today, like perfumes, fabrics, or detergents *Reflect on whether any of these might have caused dryness or itchiness.*

....

....

How did my skin respond to different environments today? *Did air conditioning, humidity, or sun exposure impact dryness or irritation?*

....

....

Have I noticed any new sensitivities or reactions lately? *Con-*

sider if any particular foods, products, or environmental factors have caused new irritation.

....

....

How does my skin feel after showering, and does water temperature seem to make a difference? *Hot water can strip oils; note if cooler showers help retain more moisture.*

....

....

6

Managing your mental and emotional health for healthy skin

It is essential to take a holistic approach to healthy skin. Mental and emotional factors can impact skin health. Taking care of your mental health can improve your overall well-being and skin health. Stress and anxiety can exacerbate symptoms such as dryness. I have compiled a list of ways to care for your skin mentally.

Sufficient sleep: During sleep, the skin cells undergo a process of repairing and regenerating. Collagen production peaks during sleep, contributing to skin elasticity, firmness, and hydration. It is essential for maintaining skin structure and preventing signs of ageing. Establish a daily sleep routine with at least 7 hours of undisturbed sleep. Create a relaxing bedtime routine and avoid staring at your screens before you sleep. Silk and satin-based or hypoallergenic bedding will be kind to the skin.

Managing Stress: Stress triggers the release of cortisol, the stress hormone. Elevated cortisol levels can increase inflammation, exacerbating skin conditions such as eczema and psoriasis. Chronic stress can weaken the skin's barrier function; a compromised skin barrier can result in dryness and dehydration. Prolonged stress can accelerate the ageing process by the breakdown of collagen.

Engage in your preferred relaxation techniques, such as meditation, yoga, deep breathing, and mindfulness. Going outdoors for fresh air, walking in the park, exercising regularly, or even having a cup of tea can help your overall well-being. Identify sources of stress in your life, such as relationships, work, or responsibilities, and take steps to address, minimise or set boundaries to protect your well-being.

Journaling and Reflection: Journal to express your thoughts, feelings, and experiences regarding your skin condition. Track your progress and reflect on your skin health to identify patterns and triggers that may affect your skin.

Self-Compassion: Be kind to yourself. Practice self-compassion by acknowledging your feelings and accepting any imperfections. Own your skin and be comfortable in it. Use daily positive affirmations to challenge negative self-talk and cultivate a positive mindset.

Self-Journal

Stress

How stressed did I feel today, and did I notice any changes in

my skin as a result Reflect on whether stress correlated with dryness, itching, or irritation.

....
....

Did I engage in any stress-relieving activities today? *Consider meditation, exercise, journaling, or spending time in nature, and note if these had a positive effect on your skin's appearance or feel?*

....
....
....
....

How does my skin feel during or after particularly stressful periods? *Look for specific changes, like increased sensitivity, flakiness, or itchiness?*

....
....
....

Are there certain situations or people that seem to stress me out more and impact my skin? *Identify any patterns between stressful interactions and your skin's health.*

....
....
....

Self-Image and Confidence

How did I feel about my skin today? *Reflect on whether you felt self-conscious, confident, or neutral about your skin's appearance.*

....

....

....

Did I avoid any activities today because of concerns about my skin? *Consider whether worries about your skin kept you from engaging in social, physical, or public activities?*

....

....

....

....

Did I practice any positive affirmations or self-acceptance exercises today? *If so, reflect on whether this helped improve your self-image and self-compassion?*

....

....

....

What compliments or positive observations did I make about my skin today? *Celebrating small wins, like a hydrated spot or smoother texture, can boost confidence*

....

....

Emotional Triggers and Skin Reactions

Did I experience any strong emotions today, and how did my skin feel afterward? *Notice if feelings like anger, sadness, or joy seem to affect your skin, even subtly?*

Are there times when my skin feels particularly dry after an emotional event or day ?*Note if certain feelings seem to impact your hydration, potentially due to physical reactions like crying or facial tension.*

Do I tend to touch or rub my skin when feeling stressed or emotional? *If so, consider if this habit may contribute to dryness or irritation?*

What positive actions can I take tomorrow if I encounter these emotional triggers *Consider strategies like deep breathing, taking* *breaks, or self-kindness to help ease stress's impact on your skin?*

....

....

....

Self-Care Practices for Emotional and Skin Health

Did I prioritise my own needs today? *Self-care is critical for both mental well-being and skin health; record if you made time for yourself?*

....

....

How did I feel after my skincare routine today? *Notice if taking time to care for your skin boosted your mood or self-esteem?*

....

....

Did I get enough sleep last night, and how did that impact my mood and skin today? *Good sleep is essential for both emotional resilience and skin repair.*

....

....

Did I set aside time for relaxation or mindfulness practices, like meditation or deep breathing? *Notice if these activities* *helped keep your stress levels in check and may have helped with dryness.*

....

....

Weekly Reflection

What were the biggest emotional triggers for my skin this week, and how did I manage them? Reflect on any patterns in your mood and skin reactions and what strategies were helpful?

....

....

....

How did I feel about my skin this week overall, and did that impact my mood or stress levels? *Look for connections between skin confidence and general emotional well-being?*

....

....

What positive mental health practices can I continue next week to support my skin? *Identify habits like daily gratitude, mindfulness, or relaxation techniques that benefit both your skin and mental health?*

....

....

....
...

What moments of self-acceptance or self-compassion did I experience this week? *Celebrate times when you felt kind toward yourself and recognise their importance in skin and mental health.*

....
....
....
...

7

Changing habits and avoiding triggers

When you have dry skin, eczema, or ichthyosis, you're walking a fine line between hydration and irritation. Your skin has a language of its own, and it doesn't speak well with harsh ingredients. Avoid the following which will further exacerbate dry skin.

Showering in hot water: Long, steamy showers might feel great, but they deplete your skin of essential moisture. Stick to lukewarm water, and your skin will be much happier.

Rough Towels: Patting dry with a soft towel so there is less friction and less irritation.

Over-Washing and Long Showers: Spending too much time in water, especially hot water, washes away the skin's protective oils, leaving it vulnerable. Keep showers brief.

Using harsh exfoliants: High-pH soaps or cleansers strip your skin's natural oils, which you want to avoid when dealing with dry skin, eczema, or ichthyosis. opt for something gentle and pH-balanced instead.

Clay-Based or Mattifying Products: e.g. Kaolin Clay, Bentonite Clay. These ingredients absorb moisture, which is great if you have oily skin. But if your skin is dry or flaky, it may make things worse by stripping away the little hydration you have left.

Alcohol-Based Ingredients. Denatured Alcohol (Alcohol Denat.): Denatured alcohol dry your skin as it evaporates hydration from your skin. It's usually found in toners.

Fragrances and Essential Oils

Synthetic Fragrances (Parfum): If your skin had a voice, it would scream at this ingredient. Fragrances smell lovely, but they are not friendly to sensitive skin, causing irritation and triggering eczema flare-ups.

Citrus Essential Oils (Lemon, Orange): Sounds refreshing, right? But on sensitive or dry skin, citrus oils can cause further irritation. They can irritate, dry, and even make your skin more vulnerable to the sun.

Strong Essential Oils (Eucalyptus, Peppermint, Tea Tree): While this sound natural and healing, for skin like yours, they're the opposite. They sting and can dry out already struggling skin, making eczema or ichthyosis even worse.

Harsh Surfactants

Sodium Lauryl Sulfate (SLS): Think of this as a moisture thief. Found in a shocking number of cleansers and body washes, it strips away your skin's natural oils like they're optional, leaving it barren. If your skin already feels like a desert, SLS is only going to turn it into a sandstorm.

Ammonium Lauryl Sulfate (ALS): This is SLS's equally bad sibling. It does the same damage, only more quietly. Don't let it sneak into your routine.

Self-Journal

Shower and Bath Habits

What temperature was my shower today? Reflect on whether it was hot, warm, or lukewarm and how your skin felt afterward.

....

....

How long did I spend in the shower today? *Notice if shorter showers leave your skin feeling less dry or irritated?*

....

....

Did I pat my skin dry with a soft towel, or did I rub it? *Note if gentle drying reduces any irritation or redness compared to rubbing.*

....

....

How does my skin feel immediately after showering? *Observe if it feels tight, itchy, or comfortable, and consider if adjustments in temperature or time might help.*

....

....

Cleansers and Exfoliants

What cleanser did I use today, and did it leave my skin feeling tight or dry? *Track if your cleanser is pH-balanced and gentle or if it might be stripping away natural oils.*

....

....

Did I use any exfoliating products today? *Notice if these left your skin red, irritated, or extra dry, and consider if they are too harsh.*

....

....

Did my skin feel any irritation or sensitivity after washing my face or body today? *Note if harsh cleansers or exfoliants could be the cause and adjust if needed.*

....

....

Am I using clay-based or mattifying products? Record any changes in skin texture or hydration if these types of products are in your routine, as they may worsen dryness.

....

....

Ingredients in Skincare Products

Did I use any products with denatured alcohol or other drying ingredients today? *Check labels for ingredients like "alcohol denat." in toners or cleansers and see if these correlate with extra dryness.*

....

....

Did I use any fragranced products today, including perfumes, scented lotions, or body washes? *Reflect on whether this causes irritation, itchiness, or dryness, and consider switching to fragrance-free options.*

....

....

Am I using any essential oils in my skincare routine? *Notice if citrus oils or strong essential oils like eucalyptus, peppermint, or tea tree leave your skin dry, tight, or sensitive?*

....

....

Did my skin feel comfortable or irritated after applying my skincare products today?*Track whether the products you're using could contain hidden irritants and adjust if needed.*

....

....

Surfactants and Foaming Cleansers

Did my cleanser contain Sodium Lauryl Sulfate (SLS) or Ammonium Lauryl Sulfate (ALS)? These can strip moisture—note any increase in dryness or discomfort.

....

....

Did I use any foaming or lathering cleansers on my skin today? Reflect on whether these products make your skin feel drier or cause flakiness?

....

....

How does my skin feel after washing with my current cleanser? Notice if it feels soft and comfortable or if it feels tight and stripped, possibly indicating harsh surfactants?

....

....

Reflecting on Triggers and Adjustments

Did I make any adjustments to my routine today to avoid dryness triggers? Consider changes in water temperature, using fragrance-free products, or choosing gentle cleansers, and observe how your skin reacts.

....

....

Have I noticed an improvement in my skin after avoiding certain ingredients? Track any positive changes in your skin when you avoid harsh chemicals and habits.

....

....

What products or habits seem to make my skin drier, and how can I replace them with gentler options? Identify patterns of irritation and explore alternatives that are hydrating and soothing

....

....

Did I feel more in control of my skin's comfort and hydration today? Reflect on the impact of being mindful about avoiding harsh products and habits and how that affected your skin.

....

....

8

Journaling skin condition

Tracking your dry skin journey can be a rewarding and enlightening experience. Here's a fresh approach to capturing your progress, experiences, and insights along the way:

Create a Skin Diary:

Daily Reflections: Dedicate a section for daily observations about your skin's condition. Note any fluctuations, flare-ups, or moments of improvement.

Routine Log: Record your skincare routine, detailing the products you use, how you apply them, and any changes you make.

Capture Visual Progress:

Before and After Photos: Take pictures of your skin at various stages to visually document your journey.

Consistent Check-Ins: Snap weekly or monthly photos in the same lighting and position to monitor how your skin evolves over time.

Identify Triggers:

Lifestyle Log: Keep track of foods, skincare products, and environmental factors that could impact your skin. This helps you pinpoint potential triggers.

Weather and Mood Correlation: Note how different weather conditions and your emotional state affect your skin, helping you identify patterns.

Evaluate Product Performance:

Usage Timeline: Log the start and stop dates for each product, along with your observations regarding their effects on your skin.

Review and Rate: Reflect on your experience with each product, noting both positive and negative reactions.

Mood and Wellness:

Emotional Influence: Write about your mood and stress levels, noting any correlation with your skin's condition. This can uncover how your mental state impacts your skin.

Self-Care Insights: Document your self-care routines and their effects on your skin and overall well-being.

Food and Hydration Record:

Nutritional Log: Keep a food diary to see if certain foods contribute to or alleviate your skin issues.

Hydration Tracker: Monitor your water intake and see if increased hydration leads to noticeable skin improvements.

Professional records:

Appointment Records: Keep a detailed account of your visits to dermatologists or skincare specialists, including their recommendations and any treatments suggested.

Post-Appointment Reflections: After each visit, jot down your thoughts on the advice received and how you plan to implement it.

Inspiration Board:

Visual Goals: Assemble a collection of inspiring images, quotes, and articles that resonate with you and embody your skin aspirations. This can serve as a motivational reminder of your journey.

Reflective Reviews:

Regular Reflection Time: Set aside moments to review your entries, photos, and patterns. Consider what strategies worked well and what didn't, allowing you to adjust your approach.

Celebrate Your Progress: Acknowledge every improvement, no matter how small, and reward yourself for your dedication to skin health.

Share Your Experience:

Social Platforms: If you feel comfortable, consider documenting your journey on social media or a blog to connect with others facing similar skin challenges. Your experiences could inspire someone else!

Join Supportive Communities: Engage with online forums or local groups where you can share your story and gain insights from others.

Documenting your dry skin journey isn't just about tracking changes; it's about gaining valuable insights, fostering a deeper understanding of your skin's needs, and celebrating the progress you make along the way. Embrace this process as a powerful tool for empowerment and self-discovery!

Self- Journal

Skin Diary

What did my skin feel like today? Note any sensations like dryness, tightness, itching, or relief.

....

....

Did I notice any significant improvements or new flare-ups? Reflect on what may have contributed to these changes.

....

....

What skincare products did I use today, and how did I apply them? Describe any variations in your routine or technique.

....

....

Visual Progress

What differences do I notice when I compare today's photo to earlier ones? Look for specific changes in texture, hydration, or areas of improvement.

....

....

Identifying Triggers

Did I eat or drink anything new today? Track if there are any correlations with flare-ups or improvements.

....

....

What were the weather conditions today, and how did my skin

respond? Note if humidity, sun exposure, or cold air affects your skin's hydration.

....

....

Was I exposed to any environmental irritants? Consider pollution, allergens, or irritants that could affect sensitive skin.

....

....

Evaluating Product Performance

How long have I been using each product in my routine? Keep a timeline to see if consistency or switching products impacts your skin.

....

....

What effects did I notice from each product today? Describe any immediate or gradual reactions, both positive and negative.

....

....

If I were to rate this product, what score would I give it and why? Identify if it's worth continuing, adjusting, or replacing.

....

....

Mood and Wellness

How did I feel emotionally today, and did it impact my skin?
Look for patterns between mood, stress levels, and skin condition.

....
....

**What self-care practices did I engage in, and how did they
make me feel?** Reflect on any mental benefits, as well as their
effect on your skin.

....
....

Did I experience any particular stressors today? Track if stress
correlates with skin changes, like itching or dryness.

....
....

Food and Hydration Record

What did I eat and drink today? Record what you consume and
note if it affects hydration or skin irritation.

....
....

How much water did I drink today, and did I notice a difference in my skin? Observe if increased hydration over time improves skin texture or reduces dryness.

....
....

Did I consume any specific food groups that seemed to help or irritate my skin? Consider the role of nutrients, sugar, dairy, or processed foods.

....
....

Professional Records

What did my dermatologist or specialist recommend today? Keep track of new treatments, products, or advice.

....
....

How do I feel about the advice I received, and how will I implement it? Reflect on any steps you plan to take or any hesitations you may have

....
....

Inspiration Board

What motivates me to take care of my skin today? Consider any goals or inspirations that keep you committed to your journey.

....

....

Are there any quotes, images, or tips that resonate with my skincare journey? Add these as reminders to stay positive and dedicated.

....

....

Reflective Reviews

What patterns have I noticed by reviewing my earlier entries? Look for trends, such as triggers or routines that work well for you.

....

....

What is one positive change in my skin over the past month? Celebrate even small improvements to boost motivation and self-appreciation.

....

....

What adjustments might I make based on my recent observations? Consider any tweaks in products, diet, or habits to further improve your skin.

....

....

Sharing Your Experience

What aspects of my journey could benefit someone else with similar skin challenges? Reflect on advice or experiences you might share in a community or support group.

....

....

What online forums, groups, or blogs inspire or encourage me? Consider joining these spaces to connect with others who understand your experience

....

....

9

Conclusion

In Conclusion, adopting a holistic approach to skincare is vital in maintaining healthy and hydrated skin. By addressing the physical, emotional, and environmental factors that impact skin health, you can create a skincare routine that nurtures and supports your skin's needs. Patience, consistency, and self-care are essential in achieving and maintaining healthy skin.

Maintaining a healthy skin routine for dry skin conditions involves embracing self-care practices, managing stress, and listening to your skin's needs. By identifying your specific type of skin condition, you can effectively target and focus on your needs with the best products and techniques.

Concluding thoughts on achieving healthy, hydrated, and glowing skin: Self-love and perseverance are essential. Embrace the lifestyle change and the journey with your skin. Celebrate the progress you make on your skincare journey and remember that healthy skin reflects your overall well-being.

My skin journey is an integral part of who I am. In the past, it felt like it overruled my life, but now I've learned to manage my ichthyosis vulgaris, and in doing so, I feel empowered and in control. Caring for my skin has become a meaningful part of my daily routine, and this dedication has shaped who I am today. Through my unique skin, I carry a piece of my grandad and family members with me, connecting us in a special way.

10

References

What is Ichthyosis. (n.d.). Ichthyosis Support Group. Retrieved November 21, 2024, from https://www.ichthyosis.org.uk/Pages/FAQs/Category/what-is-ichthyosis

Dinulos, J. G. H. (2023, May 11). *Dry skin (Xeroderma).* MSD Manual Consumer Version. https://www.msdmanuals.com/en-nz/home/skin-disorders/cornification-disorders/dry-skin-xeroderma

Tanya. (2024, July 30). Skin allergy Types and Triggers - Universal Meal Assistant. *Universal Meal Assistant - Free digital menu, calorie and nutrition tracker.* https://www.umaapp.com/skin-allergy-types-and-triggers/

Culligan, I. (2020, September 22). *Is hard or soft water better for your skin? Everything you need to know.* Ising's Culligan. https://isingsculligan.com/is-hard-or-soft-water-better-for-your-skin-everything-you-need-to-know/

Admin, & Admin. (2023, December 7). *Holistic approaches for healthy skin: from inside out.* Logical Reporter. https://logicalreporter.com/holistic-approaches-for-healthy-skin-from-inside-out/

Ames, H. (2024, June 7). *What causes menopause joint pain and what to do about it.* https://www.medicalnewstoday.com/articles/menopause-and-joint-pain#what-to-do

Website, N. (2023, May 11). *Ichthyosis.* nhs.uk. https://www.nhs.uk/conditions/ichthyosis/